No
Skid Marks

How To Clean Your Butt

No
Skid Marks

How To Clean Your Butt

By

Pat Ross

No
Skid Marks

Copyright © 2019 by Pat Ross

All Rights Reserved

Printed in the United States of America

Printing History

First Printing: December, 2019

This is a nonfiction book and all thoughts and views are based on the author's opinion only.

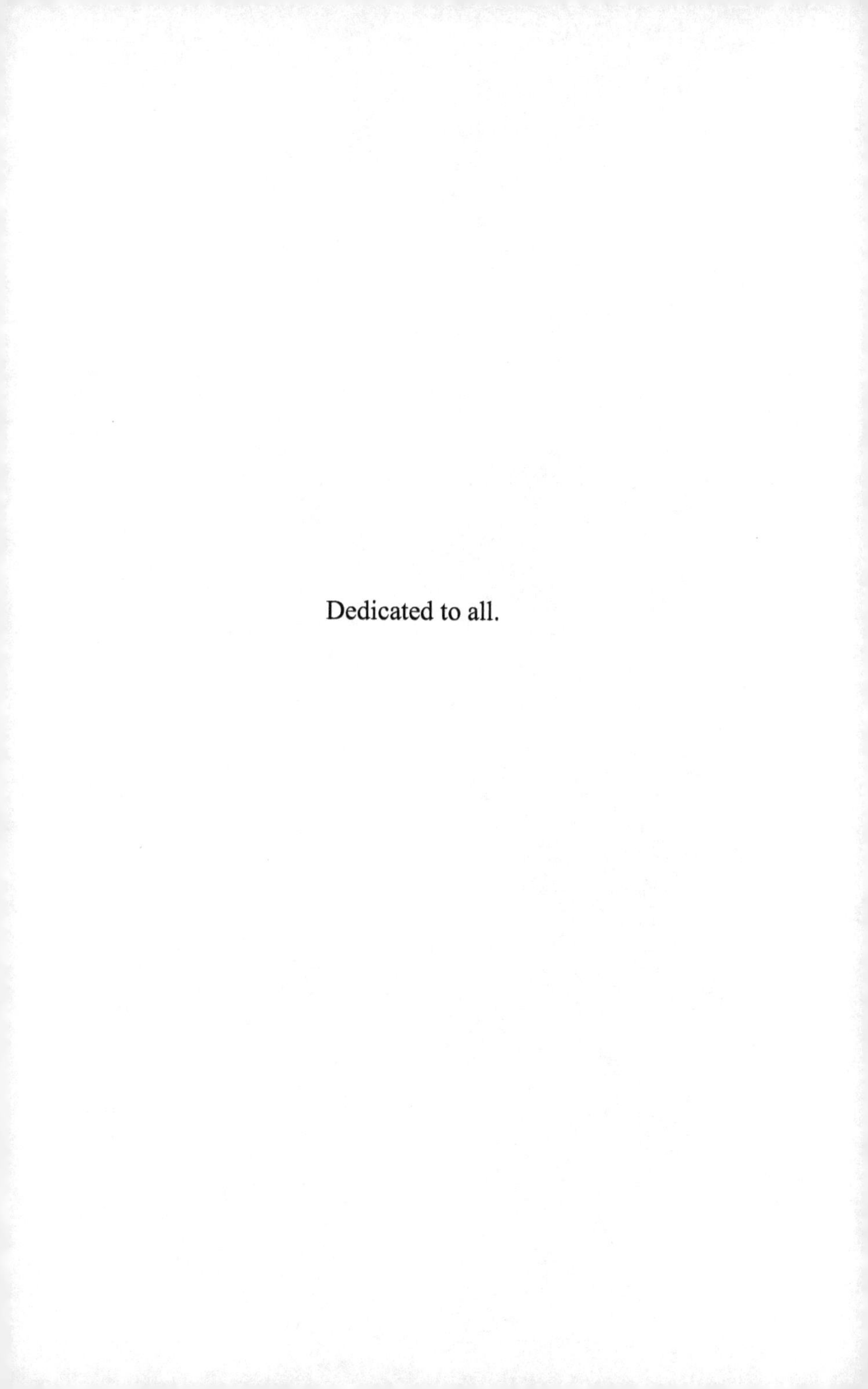

Dedicated to all.

No Skid Marks

INTRODUCTION

Surprisingly a lot of people do not properly know how to clean their butt after using the restroom. At know fault of their own no one actually taught them as a kid. Most people take this fundamental task as being self-taught or self-known and spend their adult life with the embarrassing skid marks. In this book you will learn how to rid the skid marks forever!

Pat Ross

No Skid Marks

Most people use the front to
back and reverse back to front
method for cleaning their butt.

Pat Ross

No Skid Marks

This could lead to skid marks
and wasting toilet tissue.

Pat Ross

No Skid Marks

As a kid I used this front to back and reverse back to front method and resulted in skid marks.

Pat Ross

No Skid Marks

I was so embarrassed that I
threw my underwear in the
trash before my mother would
see them in the laundry.

Pat Ross

No Skid Marks

One day I struck up the
courage to ask my mother how
to clean my butt and not have
skid marks?

Pat Ross

No Skid Marks

What she told me was eye
opening and life changing!

Pat Ross

No Skid Marks

She told me, 'you have to
pinch!"

Pat Ross

No Skid Marks

Yes. Use a rectangular portion
of toilet tissue consisting of
approximately 7 sheets.

Pat Ross

No Skid Marks

Then place the toilet tissue over
your butt hole area.

Pat Ross

No Skid Marks

Pinch the toilet tissue together
to enclose the poop.

Pat Ross

No Skid Marks

The pinching technique
contains the poop and prevents
it from moving to other places
as you wipe.

Pat Ross

No Skid Marks

Fold the toilet tissue to a clean side and repeat the pinching technique and folding as necessary.

Pat Ross

No Skid Marks

Get more toilet tissue and
repeat the previous steps until
your butt hole area is clean.

Pat Ross

No Skid Marks

For people with larger butts use your free hand to hold one of your butt cheeks open, while applying the pinching technique.

Pat Ross

No Skid Marks

Test the pinching technique and wear a pair of white underwear.

Pat Ross

No Skid Marks

Congratulations. You no
longer have skid marks!

Pat Ross

No Skid Marks

Now bravely wear that white
underwear.

Pat Ross

No Skid Marks

The End